Childhood Asthma

Childhood Asthma

What it is and what you can do

Neil Buchanan, M.D., and Peter Cooper, M.D.

Foreword by John McQuitty, M.D.

Illustrated by Jack Newnham

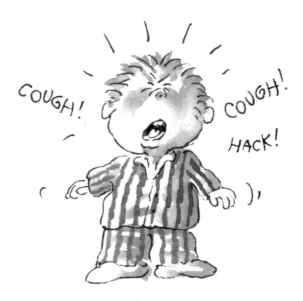

TRICYCLE PRESS
Berkeley, California

Acknowledgments

The author would like to thank those parents whose questions led to the writing of this book. I am also indebted to Professor P. Phelan, Drs. P. Van Asperen and C. Mellis, Mrs. L. Cody and Mrs. L. Adams for having read and criticized the manuscript. In addition, I am indebted to Miss K. Collison for secretarial assistance, to the audiovisual department of the Westmead Center for the illustrations, to Glaxo (Australia), Fisons Pty Ltd., and to Pitman Publishing for permission to reproduce other illustrations.

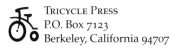 TRICYCLE PRESS
P.O. Box 7123
Berkeley, California 94707

A Kirsty Melville Book
Many thanks to Dr. John McQuitty of the Pediatric Pulmonary Unit at Children's Hospital, Oakland, California, for his review of this book.

Library of Congress Cataloging-in-Publication Data

Buchanan, Neil, PhD.
    Childhood asthma : what it is and what you can do / Neil Buchanan and Peter Cooper; illustrated by Jack Newnham; foreword by John McQuitty.
       p. cm.
    "A Kirsty Melville book".
    Includes index.
    ISBN 1-883672-36-8
    I. Cooper, Peter J.
RJ436.A8B83 1995
618.92'238—dc20   95-31279
                                         CIP

First published in Australia and New Zealand in 1991 by Doubleday
First Tricycle Press printing, 1995
Manufactured in the United States of America

1 2 3 4 5 6 — 99 98 97 96 95

Contents

Foreword

An estimated 20 percent of North American children will wheeze while growing up, and 10 percent will develop the disease characterized by wheezing called asthma. Studies show the incidence of asthma is increasing in both adults and children. In addition, these studies show the severity of asthma has increased over the last 30 years with more children requiring hospitalization and more intensified treatment in the hospital.

The authors of this book, Neil Buchanan and Peter Cooper, have been involved with treating asthma patients in a unit whose philosophy is that a well-informed patient and family are better able to cope with this disease, and to improve the quality of life for all involved. They have written this book to help parents and teachers care for children by better understanding the disease, its classification and treatment, and how it is diagnosed. *Childhood Asthma* explains asthma, what causes it, how we breathe, what triggers an attack, and answers parents' frequently asked questions. This book seeks to assure an easier life for all involved with the child who has asthma. And it succeeds because it does all of the above soundly, yet with the realization that the patient is a young child and the reader is a worried parent.

Readers may find that some of the medication names and the dosage, as well as other terms, are different than what they use with their child. For instance, Buchanan and Cooper explain asthma and its classifications as episodic, frequent attack, and chronic severe, while others have used the terms mild, moderate, and severe. However, the principles of treatment are universal, and the family who reads this book will learn much about proven treatments.

—John C. McQuitty, M.D.
Pediatric Pulmonary Center
Children's Hospital, Oakland, California

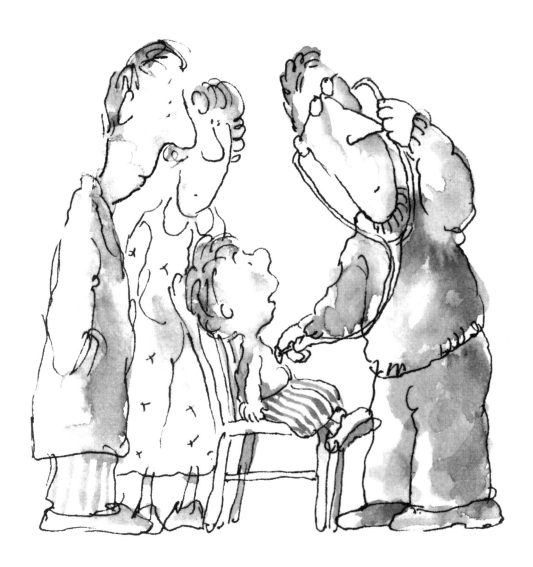

Chapter 1

What is asthma?

Asthma is a common condition which occurs in up to 20 percent of children in North America at some time or other during their childhood. This of course does not mean that 20 percent of children have asthma at any one time.

Asthma appears to be twice as common in boys as girls and boys often have more severe symptoms. This sex difference disappears in adolescence. About 30 percent of asthmatic children will have developed asthma by two years of age and about 80 percent by five years of age.

How do we breathe?

To understand asthma, it is important to have some knowledge of how we breathe and the anatomy of the lungs (how the lungs are made up). We breathe in air through the nose and mouth, and the lining (mucosa) of these areas is warm and moist. This means the air we breathe in is warmed and moistened before it reaches the lungs. In addition, dust particles stick to the mucosa rather than being sucked into the lungs. Once the air has reached the back of the throat, it goes through the larynx (voice box) into the lungs.

The lungs are made up of the main airway, the trachea, which divides into two main airways (bronchi), the left and right main bronchus, which go to the left and right lungs, respectively. These main bronchi then subdivide many times into smaller airways (bronchioles) with each bronchiole ending up in a little balloon-like sac called an alveolus. Air comes down the trachea, into the bronchi, bronchioles and lastly into the alveoli. In the alveoli, which have a very thin lining, oxygen from the air crosses the lining and goes into the bloodstream. At the same time, the gas we breathe out, carbon dioxide, crosses the alveolar lining in the opposite direction, from the bloodstream to the alveolus. So we breathe in oxygen and breathe out (exhale) carbon dioxide.

Before discussing what asthma is, it is important to know a little more about the bronchi, their structure and function. The bronchi have three layers:

- An outer layer of incomplete rings of cartilage. This makes the bronchus stiff and maintains its shape;

- A middle, circular layer of smooth muscle which by contracting and relaxing alters the size of the bronchus;

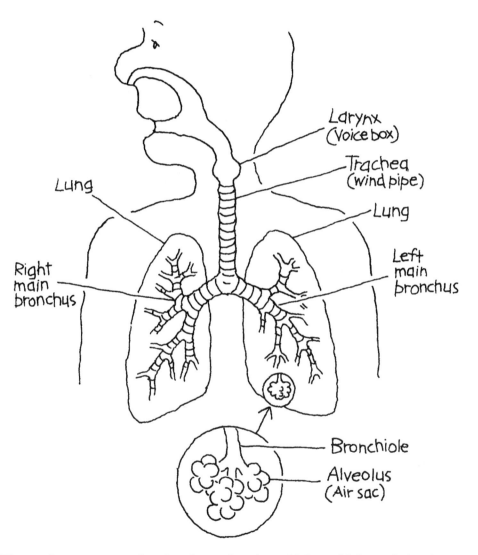

The respiratory system showing the trachea, bronchi, bronchioles and alveoli.

• An inner layer of mucosa (lining) which consists of mucus, mucus-producing glands and little hairs called cilia.

Mucus is being produced all the time and traps dust and other particles. It is swept upwards to the back of the throat by the cilia and is then swallowed. This goes on all the time and we are unaware of it.

What happens in asthma?

All airways are reactive; in other words, any of us when exposed to smoke as in a fire or to a lot of dust, will cough and splutter. This is because the lining of the airways, the mucosa, is irritated and produces more mucus and this needs to be coughed up. In people with asthma, the airways are hyper-reactive, in other words, unusually sensitive to outside irritants. This means that irritants such as dust, pollens, etc., which would not affect most people, produce an excessive (hyper-reactive) response in the asthmatic.

In this situation three main things occur in the bronchi. There is excessive production of mucus, swelling of the lining of the airway, tightening (constriction) of the smooth muscle. The end result of these events is that the lumen (center) of the bronchus is narrowed. This makes the passage of air difficult and results in wheezing and trouble with breathing. When the narrowing is less severe, coughing may be the only symptom of asthma. So the basic problem in asthma is that the airways are narrowed.

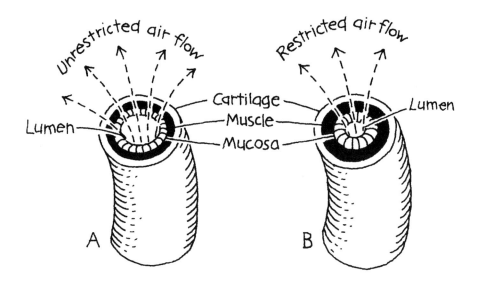

A bronchus seen end on, as if looking down a tube. The passage in the middle of the bronchus is called the lumen. (A) is the normal bronchus. (B) is the bronchus in asthma with the muscle contracted, the mucosa swollen and the lumen narrowed.

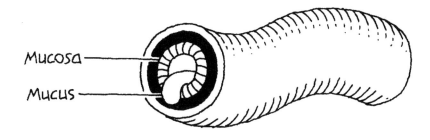

Mucus secretion provokes coughing.

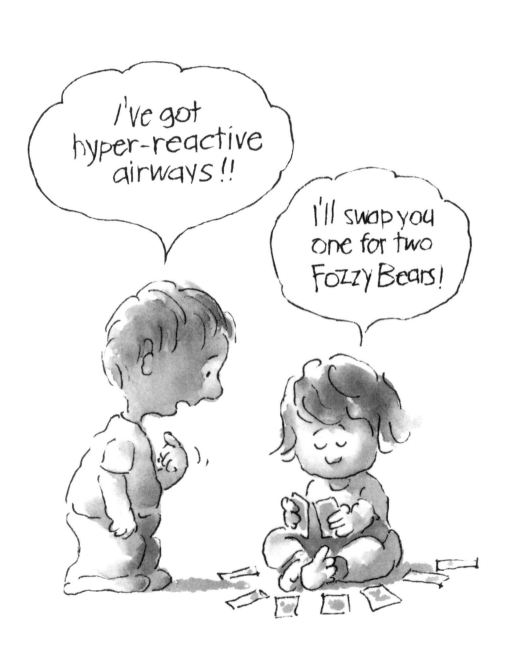

Chapter 2

What causes asthma?

There are numerous causes of asthma, some more important in one person than in others.

The first point to bear in mind is that asthma occurs in people predisposed to the condition; in other words, those with hyper-reactive airways. Bronchial hyper-reactivity may be inherited as it can be induced in symptom-free relatives of asthmatic children and is much commoner in identical than non-identical twins. It is against this background of hyper-reactivity that the agents precipitating asthma act.

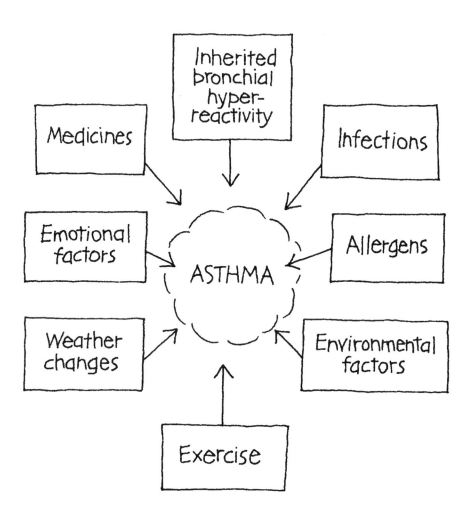

The causes of asthma.

Infections

The commonest cause of an attack of asthma is a viral infection. Many parents will notice their child develops a cold, runny nose and then starts coughing. This may be followed by wheezing over the next day or two. Why such infections provoke asthma is uncertain, but it is thought that they stimulate the hyper-reactive airways to narrow. These infections are almost invariably due to viruses, which do not respond to antibiotics. So antibiotics are very rarely needed in the management of an acute episode of asthma. Viral infections are most common in late autumn and winter, so childhood asthma is particularly common during these seasons.

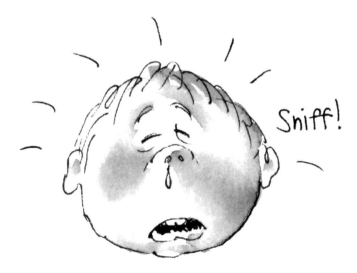

Allergic factors

Asthma can be induced by agents to which the child is allergic. These are called allergens and include:

■ Pollens

Pollens are carried in the wind and are inhaled. They may arise from trees, grasses or flowers and differ in various parts of the world. Pollens are only around during pollination which is usually only a month or so each year. They are obviously very difficult allergens to avoid.

■ Mold

Molds, which are members of the fungus family, are widespread. They are also carried around in the air. They are usually around in the warmer months but can cause allergic symptoms indoors in the winter. High levels of molds occur in damp conditions such as rain and fog where they may be present in a damp room or in food storage areas, garbage cans, wallpaper, upholstery, etc.

■ House dust

House dust is made up of lots of components: big particles and small particles. Anyone cleaning out a dusty room will cough and sneeze, but the asthmatic with his/her sensitive bronchi may well wheeze. House dust consists of pollens, hairs and skin scales from the family pet, fragments of clothing and upholstery, dead insects and bacteria, animal and plant fibers, food remnants, etc.

Obviously it is not possible to protect oneself from all these normal things; however in practical terms, it is wise for the bedroom of an asthmatic child to be vacuumed and equipped with non-upholstered furniture, if that is possible. A foam mattress and pillow are preferable to avoid the dust in standard mattresses and pillows.

The main cause of house dust allergy is the house dust mite. Mites live on human skin and are shed with the old skin scales onto the clothes or bedding. Mites flourish in damp, temperate places and are best kept under control by keeping the dust content of the home down and ensuring that it is as well heated and ventilated as possible.

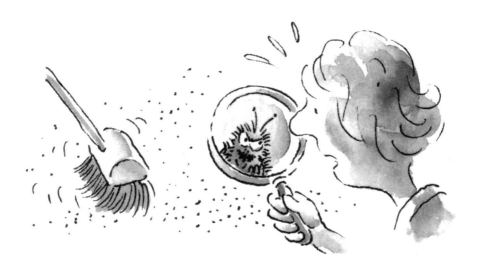

■ Pets

The fur, or sometimes the skin, scales or saliva, of a pet dog or cat may also act as an allergen. Bird feathers and the fur of other animals may also have the same effect. While the pet is around, the symptoms will persist. If you are unsure if the pet is responsible for the problems, before giving it away, try asking someone to look after it for a month or so and see if the symptoms disappear.

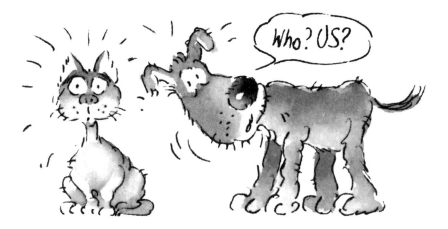

■ Food

Much has been said and written about food allergy, not only in the context of asthma but also in hay fever, feeding problems, hyperactivity and so on. Asthma is rarely caused by food allergies. Food allergy, when it occurs, is usually manifest by swollen lips and tongue, sometimes by a rash and tummy pains, and may be associated with coughing and wheezing. In other words, it is quite a dramatic event and usually the parents associate the symptoms with the food just taken by the child. If this does occur, that food should be avoided.

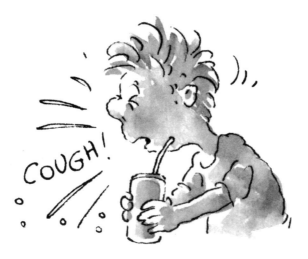

There are some preservatives in foods and soft drinks—tartrazine, sodium metabisulfite and monosodium glutamate (MSG)—which can cause problems. (See Appendix 1 for foods containing these preservatives.) Sodium metabisulfite is used to preserve soft drinks and is broken down to the irritant gas sulfur dioxide. What usually happens is that with the first drink from the bottle or can the child has a bout of coughing which may be associated with wheezing. This is a reflex response to the irritating sulfur dioxide. Children with these symptoms should avoid the offending soft drink. The effects of sodium metabisulfite, MSG or tartrazine are not related to allergy, they are a direct effect of the chemical.

Environmental factors

The environment that we live in, especially in cities, is polluted with fumes and other substances, all of which can probably precipitate an attack of asthma. Cigarette smoke can also do this either

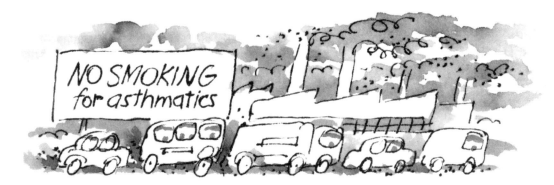

for the person smoking the cigarette or for those inhaling the 'second-hand' smoke. For children whose parents do not smoke, the incidence of asthma is 1.5 percent; where one parent smokes it rises to 4.5 percent; and if both parents smoke, the chances double that a child's asthma will worsen. Ideally parents of asthmatic children should not smoke.

Emotional factors

This is a slightly confused area and folklore suggests that asthmatic children are 'nervous' children. This is untrue. However, it is accepted that emotional upsets, excitement or disappointment can precipitate or aggravate an asthma attack. There is no particular personality type associated with asthma.

Medicines

Very few medicines given in childhood provoke an attack of asthma. The main group of medicines that may do this are called beta blockers and are very rarely used in childhood. Aspirin may also induce asthma in aspirin-sensitive patients and is best avoided.

Exercise

Some children may develop an attack of asthma during or usually after moderate or strenuous exercise, such as running around outside or participating in an organized sport such as football. This is called 'exercise-induced' asthma. It is important that parents recognize this particular form of asthma in their child, if it occurs, as it can be almost totally prevented by appropriate medication, such as the use of a puffer or Spinhaler, before exercise.

Changes in the weather

Rapid climatic changes from hot to cold, or the other way around, can precipitate an attack of asthma. Some children are worse in damp weather, while others who are allergic to grasses are more likely to have attacks in dry weather.

As can be seen there are many factors which precipitate asthma in a susceptible person. Some can be dealt with or avoided quite easily, such as exercise; others, like our environment, are almost impossible to avoid.

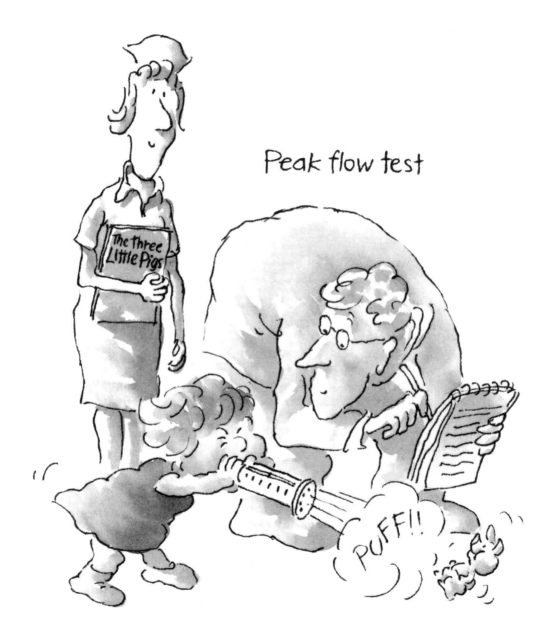

Peak flow test

Chapter 3

How is asthma diagnosed?

Asthma is diagnosed in three ways. First, from the story given by the parents of recurrent cough, wheeze or multiple episodes of so-called bronchitis. Secondly, by observations made on examination of the child, and thirdly, by a number of tests (see the table on page 27). Most children will need very few tests to make the diagnosis of asthma.

History

It is important that parents and the child give the doctor as accurate an history as possible. Attention should be paid to times at which wheezing or coughing occurs, factors which may provoke these episodes, how long they last and if they are related to exercise. Your doctor will also ask if other members of the family have asthma, hay fever or eczema. These three conditions all have an 'allergic' or 'atopic' basis and as bronchial hyper-reactivity is partly inherited, this information will help in making the diagnosis.

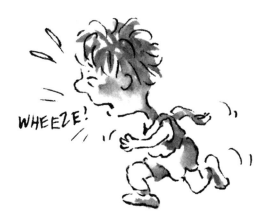

WHEEZE!

History	Recurrent cough
	Wheezing
	Breathlessness
	Breathlessness with exercise
Examination	Eczema*
	Signs of hay fever
	Wheeze
Tests	Pulmonary function tests
	Response to bronchodilators
	Exercise provocation
	Skin tests**
	RAST tests**
	Chest x-ray
	Trial of medication**

Steps in the diagnosis of asthma
  *These features may be seen in some children with asthma.
**These tests are not often required in childhood.

Examination

Many children will be quite well when they visit the doctor and nothing will be found on examination. In an acute attack, they will be wheezing and in chronic severe cases there may be a barrel chest deformity. This means that the chest is more circular ('barrel-like') than usual, due to air trapped in the lungs chronically because of the difficulty breathing out—the hallmark of asthma.

Tests

The basic test to diagnose asthma is called a 'lung (pulmonary) function' test. There are a number of ways in which this can be done. As the main problem in asthma is breathing out (expiration), the patient is asked to blow into a machine to see how well he or she can breathe out (exhale). The simplest version of this test is the 'peak flow' test. Young children, less than six to seven years of age, may not be able to cooperate sufficiently to do these tests.

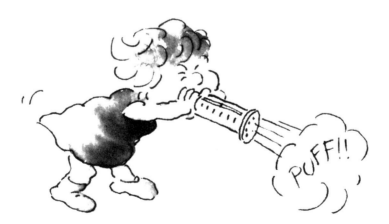

■ Pulmonary function tests

As mentioned above, the child would be asked to blow into a peak flow meter or perhaps a more sophisticated device. This is like blowing into a balloon. The child's performance over three or four blows would be compared to known normal values for his or her age and size. If peak flow is diminished this supports the diagnosis of asthma. It should be remembered that asthma comes and goes and when the child has the test done he or she may be quite well and the test normal. A normal peak flow at one particular time does not exclude asthmas. Your doctor may ask you to monitor your child's breathing at home with such a device.

■ Response to bronchodilators

To go one step further, in a patient in whom a low peak flow has been demonstrated, a bronchodilator (a medication which dilates and widens the bronchi) can be given and the test repeated. In general, a medication such as albuteral (Ventolin) or terbutaline sulfate (Bricanyl) would be given by nebulizer and the test repeated in ten minutes. An improvement in peak flow of 15–20 percent means that the bronchi have responded to the medication and this also strongly supports the diagnosis of asthma.

■ Exercise provocation

Another way of making the diagnosis, especially in children with exercise-induced asthma, is to do a peak flow test before and after exercise in order to demonstrate a fall in peak flow. The next step is to give some medication before the exercise and to show that it stops, or at least decreases, the previously demonstrated fall in peak flow. In some patients, it may be necessary to give either histamine or metacholine which will produce a fall in peak flow in those who are asthmatic.

■ Skin tests

These are done to define the cause of the patient's allergy. A small amount of allergen extract (pollen, cat fur, etc.) is placed on the skin which is then pricked gently. If the patient is allergic to a particular allergen, a small itchy swelling will appear. These tests are not entirely reliable and do not always match up with what the patient or the parents identify as the allergen. The other problem is that in some patients there are multiple allergies about which nothing can be done. Skin tests are rarely done in children and should be restricted to very specific situations.

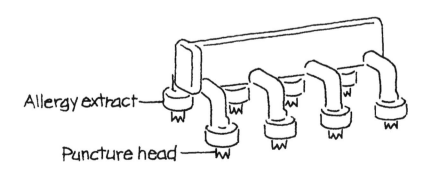

Allergy extract

Puncture head

■ RAST tests

This is a blood test to identify allergens. It is a relatively new test and therefore quite fashionable if rather expensive. Its role in the management of childhood asthma is extremely limited and has no benefit over skin tests.

■ Chest x-ray

The chest x-ray can help in the diagnosis of asthma but should only be done when necessary. There is a tendency to do a chest x-ray every time an asthmatic gets sick or is admitted to the hospital, which is quite unnecessary. The chest x-ray may show evidence of air trapping, as the patient has trouble breathing out, and because of the thick mucus produced in some patients with asthma, there may be some bronchi which are blocked. The lung beyond may also become deflated (airless) and then collapse (atelectasis). This is quite common in asthma and can be mistaken for areas of infection. In general, atelectasis will respond to breathing exercises and physiotherapy; antibiotics are not needed.

■ Trial of medication

In some patients, especially those with recurrent cough and no wheeze, it may be wise to give some bronchodilator medication for a month or so. If the symptoms disappear, then the diagnosis is asthma.

In summary, asthma can usually be diagnosed quite simply with a very limited number of tests. *Remember that a recurrent cough may, in some children, be the only symptom of asthma.*

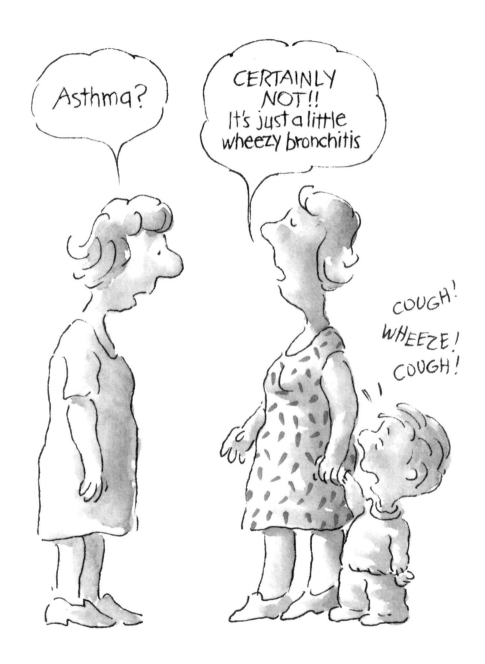

Chapter 4

What happens to children with asthma?

Broadly speaking, asthmatic children can be divided into three groups. The divisions are somewhat artificial but are useful for explaining what happens to children with asthma.

Episodic asthma

About three quarters of the children who have asthma have acute episodes or attacks which are intermittent. The episodes vary in length and severity, but lung function returns to normal between attacks. About 50 percent of these children will stop wheezing before adulthood. As far as treatment is concerned, these children only require medication for their isolated episodes of asthma, i.e., intermittent or episodic treatment.

Frequent attacks of asthma

Just under a quarter of asthmatic children have more frequent and prolonged wheezing. Their asthma usually starts in a fashion similar to the episodic group, often at a younger age. In many of these children pulmonary function tests, such as peak flow, are abnormal between attacks. Of this group about half continue to have frequent episodes in adult life, a quarter have mild asthma throughout life, and the remaining quarter grow out of it. These children who have more severe asthma and abnormal pulmonary function between attacks require regular medication, i.e., maintenance treatment. It can sometimes be difficult to decide when a child warrants maintenance treatment and this often needs to be talked about with the patient, the parents and the doctor.

Chronic severe asthma

Fortunately this is a very small proportion (1–3 percent) of all children with asthma. Four out of five such children are boys. Symptoms usually start before the age of two and often there is associated eczema and rhinitis or hay fever. All these children have

The different types of asthma in childhood. Most children have mild episodic asthma.

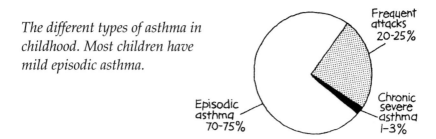

abnormal pulmonary function between attacks and in most of these children asthma continues into adult life.

For the majority of children, asthma is a mild episodic problem which responds well to fairly simple treatments. It is important to bear this in mind as for a long time the word 'asthma' has suggested to parents and doctors alike a sinister chronic condition. This is not the case at all. Unfortunately this attitude still exists as was demonstrated in a study of asthmatic children in Newcastle upon Tyne, Australia, in 1983. In a very large proportion of children with wheeze, the diagnosis of asthma had not been mentioned by the doctor. Of 176 children with wheeze, 21 were told they had asthma, 18 were told they had wheezy bronchitis or a 'chest allergy,' 126 had nonspecific diagnoses and 14 had never been seen by a doctor.

There is no purpose in avoiding the term asthma. It is much better to say 'Your child has asthma' and then spend time explaining that it is almost surely of the mild episodic type and that with time he or she will grow out of it. Without this approach these children may have continued episodes of ill health quite unnecessarily and go from one episode of so-called 'wheezy bronchitis' to the next. Children who grow out of asthma continue to have hyper-reactive airways, but without symptoms, unless they are exposed to triggering factors. Therefore they should, for example, be discouraged from ever smoking.

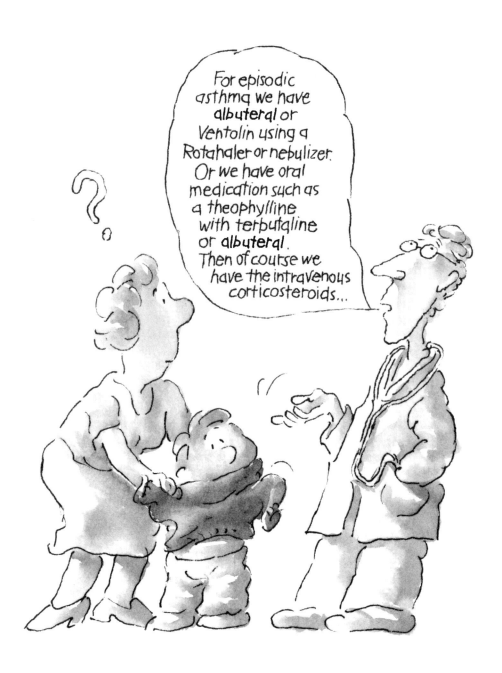

Chapter 5

How is asthma treated?

As mentioned previously, in most children asthma can be treated quite simply using a variety of medications. In this chapter we are going to first look at the forms of treatment available for the various degrees of severity of asthma and secondly examine additional treatment such as physiotherapy, breathing exercises, etc.

Episodic asthma

Episodic asthma (sometimes called mild) means that the child has infrequent attacks (episodes) of asthma. By infrequent, the doctor usually means episodes occurring less often than once a month, with few symptoms in between. He or she does not need to be on regular treatment between attacks and only needs to be treated when an attack occurs. This is called interval treatment; in other words, the child is treated at intervals when he or she is unwell, usually with short-acting reliever medications such as albuteral or terbutaline. Medication is started early (as soon as the symptoms begin) and should be continued regularly until they ease.

Episodic attacks can be treated in a number of ways depending upon their severity:

■ Inhaled medication

This is the most effective route for the initial treatment of attacks of any severity and medication can be given either using a puffer, Rotahaler, spacer (AeroChamber, Inspirease) or a nebulizer. The child inhales the medication, such as albuteral (Ventolin), and it reaches the bronchi directly where it has its effect. This form of treatment can be given up to four hourly for a few days if necessary but should not be given more frequently without a doctor being involved.

■ Medication by mouth

In mild attacks of asthma, good results may be obtained from oral (by mouth) medication. This can either be a theophylline-containing product such as TheoDur or other agents such as albuteral (Ventolin) or terbutaline sulfate (Bricanyl). These medications need to be given three to four times a day until the attack is over.

■ Intravenous treatment

Some children with episodic asthma, despite the fact that they have few attacks, may have severe episodes. These children should be treated as outlined above. If there is no improvement over 24–48 hours and especially if they get worse, they should see their doctor or go to the hospital. They may need additional treatment such as oral corticosteroids (prednisone) or oxygen. In very severe attacks, an intravenous drip containing corticosteroids and aminophylline may be necessary.

Discuss with your doctor the most appropriate method for your child.

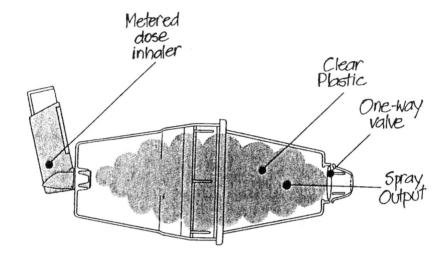

A spacer device (such as AeroChamber) suitable for delivering medica-tion to younger children (ages two upwards). The recommended dose is delivered into the device and the drug is inhaled through the one-way valve over five to ten seconds.

Age (years)	Recommended device	Medication available for device
0–2+	Nebulizer	Ventolin, Bricanyl, Atrovent, Intal
1–2+	AeroChamber with mask	Any puffer
2–5+	Spacer (with puffer): AeroChamber, Inspirease	Bricanyl, Intal, Ventolin, Beclovent
4–7+	Rotahaler Spinhaler Turbuhaler	Beclovent, Ventolin Intal Bricanyl
7+	Metered dose aerosol: Puffer	Ventolin, Bricanyl, Atrovent, Intal

Note: Some children are able to use devices at younger ages than those shown, and certain devices, such as the nebulizer, can be used at any age.

Correct puffer technique

1. Remove the dustcap from the mouthpiece (a) and shake the inhaler vigorously.

2. Hold the inhaler vertically by either of the illustrated methods (b) (c). Breathe out slowly and gently until the lungs are comfortably empty (d).

3. Tilt the head back. Close your lips around the mouthpiece (e). As you slowly start to breathe in, press the metal canister down firmly. Continue to breathe in deeply.

4. Remove the inhaler from your mouth while holding your breath for as long as is comfortable (approximately ten seconds). This allows the medication to settle into the lower airways (f). Breathe out gently.

5. If further inhalation is required, wait for at least one minute, then repeat steps 2 to 4.

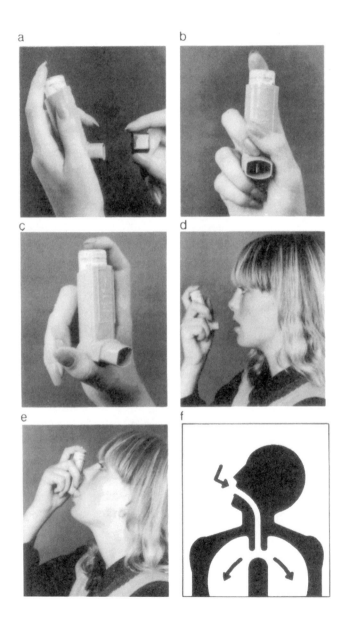

How to use a puffer inhaler. Children from age six to seven years can usually manage a puffer effectively.

Using the Rotahaler

1. With the light-blue body uppermost (vertical), hold the Rotahaler by the dark-blue mouthpiece. With the other hand turn the light-blue body as far as it will go in either direction (a).

2. Remove a Ventolin Rotacap from its foil and push it firmly, clear end first, into the raised 'square' hole so that the tip of the Rotacap's blue end is flush with the raised 'square' hole (b). This will force any previously used Rotacap shell into the Rotahaler. (Note: When first using or after washing the Rotahaler the raised 'square' hole will be empty.)

3. Holding the Rotahaler level (horizontal), turn the light-blue body with a firm movement as far as it will go in the opposite direction to open the Rotacap (c). It is essential that you keep the Rotahaler horizontal until you have inhaled the dose, as turning it upright will cause the contents of the Rotacap to fall out.
   Your Ventolin Rotahaler is now ready for use.
   Breathe out until you are comfortably empty.

4. Keeping the Rotahaler level, raise it to your mouth. Grip the dark-blue mouthpiece between your teeth and lips and tilt your head slightly backwards (d). Breathe in as strongly and as deeply as you can. Hold your breath and remove the Rotahaler from your mouth. Continue holding your breath for as long as is comfortable before gently breathing out.

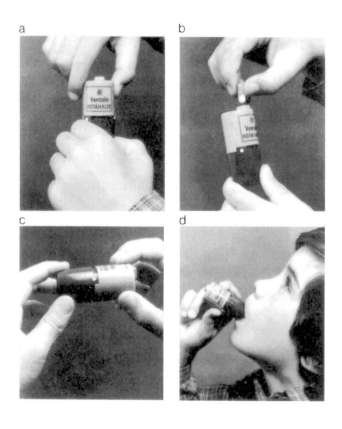

Using the Rotahaler. Most children from age four years upwards can use a Rotahaler effectively.

Frequent attacks

Children who have frequent attacks of asthma will need more active treatment. It is difficult to specify when a child is having 'frequent' attacks but doctors think of 'frequent' as meaning approximately one or more attacks a month, usually involving a few days of illness.

All of these children will have had interval treatment with reliever drugs already. Once the attacks become frequent it is preferable to use a preventative drug rather than regular reliever medications.

A child with frequent attacks needs maintenance (preventative) treatment. In other words, keeping the child on regular treatment to try and reduce the frequency of the attacks. This can be done with a number of medications:

■ Inhaled medications

The inhaled route is the most effective for maintenance treatment. Some young children, and some parents, like to use their home nebulizer two to three times a day for this purpose. In older children, the use of the puffer is more acceptable. Dry powder capsule inhalers (Spinhaler, Rotahaler) and large volume spacers (AeroChamber, Inspirease) can also be very useful ways of giving maintenance medication.

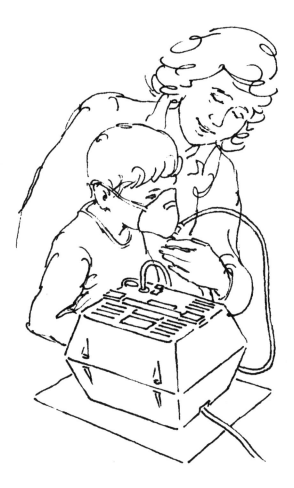

Nebulizers are necessary for delivering both reliever and preventative medications to infants and young children. They are also useful in relieving acute attacks in children of all ages. However, not every child needs a nebulizer, especially if he/she is not prone to bad attacks. Milder attacks can be managed with other devices such as a puffer or Rotahaler alone, or puffer with a large volume spacer (see page 40).

Maintenance (preventative) medications

The mainstays of treatment are:

1. Sodium cromoglycate (Intal). This is inhaled through a nebulizer, Spinhaler or puffer and needs to be given regularly 3 or 4 times a day. It is used to prevent frequent episodes of less severe asthma and can also be used, before exercising, in children with exercise-induced asthma. It is of no use in acute attacks. It is a preventative drug, not a treating (reliever) drug. It is often the first drug used in the prevention of asthma and is very helpful in the milder asthmatic. The preventative effect of Intal takes a few days to build up and a proper trial of the drug should last 4 to 6 weeks.

2. Inhaled corticosteroids (Beclovent). These are inhaled through Rotahalers, puffers and, hopefully soon, via nebulizers. They prevent more severe, frequent episodes than Intal and are often substituted when Intal has not been successful. They can be given 2, 3 or 4 times a day depending upon the severity of the asthma. Side effects are minimal with standard doses. The minimum dose that controls the symptoms is used. Higher doses are sometimes used to get a difficult situation under control and then the drug is cut back to a lower maintenance dose.

3. In addition, certain other drugs may sometimes be used as preventative agents. Examples include slow-release theophylline preparations (TheoDur) which only need to be given twice daily. For younger children, IneoDur sprinkles are also available.

Bronchodilator drugs like albuteral (Ventolin), terbutaline sulfate (Bricanyl) or orciprenaline sulfate (Alupent) help to dilate the bronchi and may sometimes be used in combination with Intal and Beclovent in maintenance treatment. However, their main use is as 'reliever' medications, given in short bursts, to stop acute interval symptoms that may break through the preventative medications.

How long a child should remain on maintenance treatment is an individual decision. Some children need treatment in the winter months only, others for the better part of the year. If your child has been taking medication for a while and is symptom-free, the only way you will know if he or she still needs more medication is by either doing lung function tests or reducing or stopping the medication. You should discuss this with your general practitioner or pediatrician.

Sodium cromoglycate (Intal) can be inhaled using a Spinhaler or puffer. With the Spinhaler, the patient breathes out and then inhales from the device. Most asthmatics will need to inhale twice

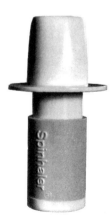

to empty the capsule. If your child needs more than three sucks to empty the capsule, then he or she may not be old, or mature, enough to use the device. If so, other methods such as a nebulizer or puffer with spacer should be tried. The correct puffer inhalation technique is shown on pages 42–43.

Sodium cromoglycate (Intal) is inhaled using a Spinhaler (above) or puffer.

■ Measuring the response to treatment (the peak flow meter)

By regularly measuring peak flows and recording readings (usually twice daily) on a chart, it is possible to detect signs of deterioration or improvement in a child's condition. It can be very useful during acute attacks, when measurements should be taken more frequently, as part of a 'crisis plan' (see Appendix 3). Monitoring shows how effectively the prescribed medication is controlling the asthma and identifies when there is a need for extra treatment.

Who needs a peak flow meter?

Not everyone with asthma needs a peak flow meter but parents often find them both helpful and reassuring. Generally, children over five who need regular therapy for frequent or chronic asthma symptoms and those who get severe attacks are most likely to benefit from home peak flow monitoring.

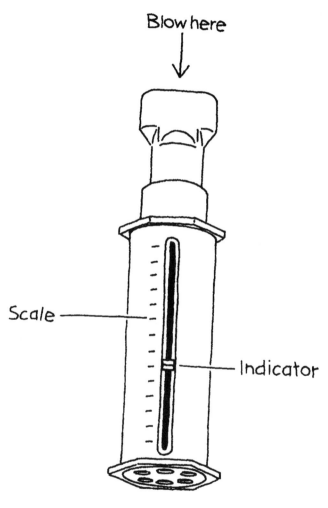

Peak flow meter

Chronic severe asthma

As we have said, this is a small group of asthmatic children (1 to 3 percent). However, for these children activities can be limited and life can be difficult. They will need all the forms of treatment that we have discussed and will have to be on very regular medication, usually inhaled steroids. In addition they may need an extra short course of steroids (prednisone) to shorten severe attacks. These children should be under the supervision of a pediatrician or a pediatric chest specialist.

They are likely to have a number of hospital admissions and need fairly constant medical guidance. They also need to be encouraged to lead as active a life as possible, to be independent and to have an understanding of their disease and its treatment.

Other forms of treatment which may occasionally be used in association with those described include:

■ Desensitization (allergy vaccines)

This form of treatment remains of *unproven value* in childhood asthma. For it to be successful, it is necessary to have identified a single, specific allergen by skin prick or RAST tests. They are rarely used in children and on occasion can cause a severe attack of asthma.

■ Antihistamines

The medicines are used to relieve some of the swelling of the mucosa. There are many antihistamines available, some of which are Actifed, Atarax, Benadryl, Periactin, Phenergan, Polaramine. Side effects of drowsiness, lack of concentration, nightmares and sometimes hyperactivity may all occur. The newer, non-sedating antihistamines such as astemizole (Hismanal) and terfenadine

(Seldane) are better for children. They have little role to play in the management of asthma, but may be of use if the patient has hay fever or eczema.

■ Cough mixtures

Most of these mixtures contain codeine or one of its derivatives and decrease the cough reflex. They are of no help in the relief of asthma.

■ Mucolytics

These are medicines such as Mucomyst that are meant to allow the bronchial mucus to be coughed up more easily. They appear to be of little, if any, use in asthmatic children.

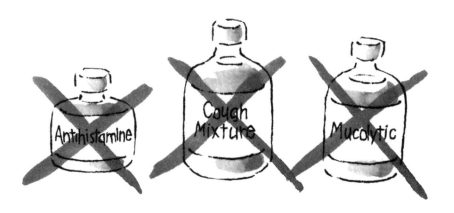

■ Physiotherapy and breathing exercises

Swimming is a useful sport for asthmatic children and allows them to become physically fitter, to relax and to control their breathing. Children with exercise-induced asthma should have an inhalation from a puffer followed by an inhalation from a Ventolin Rotahaler before starting their exercise. An alternative is to have an inhaled dose of sodium cromoglycate (Intal).

Physiotherapy can be of help to children with asthma in a number of ways:

1. Improving muscle power and getting the child in better shape.

2. Teaching the child to control breathing in a more relaxed way.

3. Encouraging good posture to improve breathing.

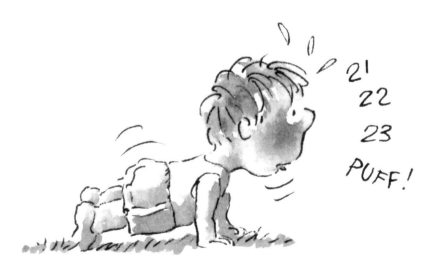

Formal physiotherapy should be for a short period of time and act as encouragement for the child to get involved in normal physical activity. Active children do their own physiotherapy.

■ Psychological support

A lot of the psychological problems suffered by asthmatic children relate to the fact that they feel themselves to be different from their peers. They may feel anxious about having attacks and not being able to participate in normal activities and may even become introverted and withdrawn because of their asthma. This is best tackled with good maintenance therapy, positive thinking and support from parents, schoolteachers, health professionals and others. These children need to be realistically encouraged to get out and about and do as much as they can. After one or two successes, a lot of the problems will be resolved.

Asthma holiday camps are also useful in encouraging independence and achievement. They provide an opportunity for kids with asthma to be together and involved in activities and exercise under supervision. They are mainly good fun and are designed to boost confidence. Ask your doctor or local Asthma Foundation or Lung Association for information about these.

■ Non-medical treatments

Parents often ask about the value of acupuncture, iridology, naturopathy or negative ion generators in the treatment of asthma. The attraction of these forms of therapy is that they are drug-free. While none of these forms of treatment is specific for asthma, they also appear to be harmless. They are however of no use in acute attacks.

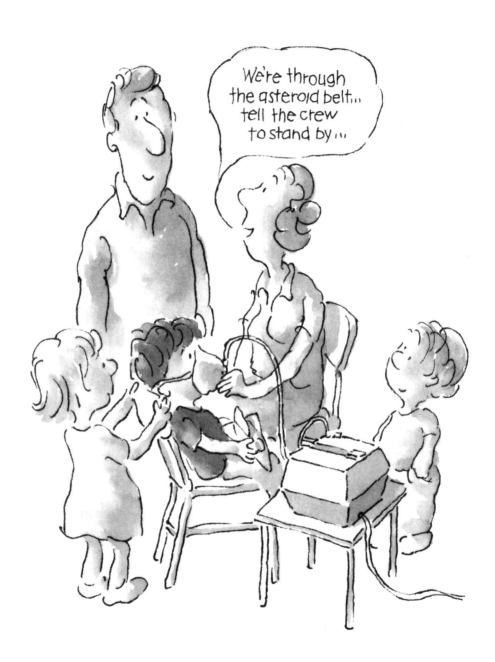

Chapter 6

What to do during an attack

Most children with asthma will have an acute attack from time to time. This is distressing for the child and the parents. It is important to know what to do when this occurs. It is also very valuable to have a written action or 'crisis' plan (see Appendix 3).

Stay calm

The more anxious and tense the child and the parents are, the worse the attack may be. If you as parents know about the medications, how to use them and if you have a written plan of action for dealing with acute attacks of asthma, things will go smoothly. Your confidence will be recognized by your child and this will be very helpful to him or her.

Medicines for the acute attack

The most useful medications are the *treating* (reliever) ones given by inhalation, namely bronchodilators such as Ventolin, Bricanyl or Alupent. These should be given by puffer, Rotahaler, spacer, or perhaps most effectively, by nebulizer. At the same time, medication can be given by mouth, but this will not have an effect for 30 to 60 minutes.

The inhaled medicines can be given up to every three to four hours at home. If this is not having any effect, then you should consult your doctor or take the child to the hospital. When you contact your doctor, explain *precisely* what you have done so far. For example: 'John began wheezing last night and I started the nebulizer right away. He has been on the machine every four hours since then and he has also had two doses of oral TheoDur. Despite this, he isn't any better . . .' This will give your doctor an idea of the severity of the attack.

Reasons to contact your doctor or to go to the hospital

Parents may sometimes find it difficult to know if their child is getting better or not. This is more difficult if your child has only recently developed asthma but is easier as time goes by and parents get more experience in managing acute episodes of asthma. If in doubt, contact your doctor or go to the hospital. Some pointers for seeking help are:

- Having to use the nebulizer more often than every three to four hours.

- If the child seems to be getting unduly tired.

- If the child shows blueness of the lips and tongue (called cyanosis). This is an emergency.

- If there is little wheezing but the child is obviously still distressed. (In severe asthma, there may be little wheeze.)

Do not be embarrassed by calling your doctor or going to the hospital if you feel uncertain about how things are going. It may be better for the child and for the parents if the child is admitted overnight just to get the attack under control. Most hospital admissions for asthma are only for two to three days.

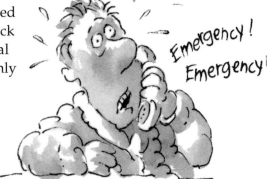

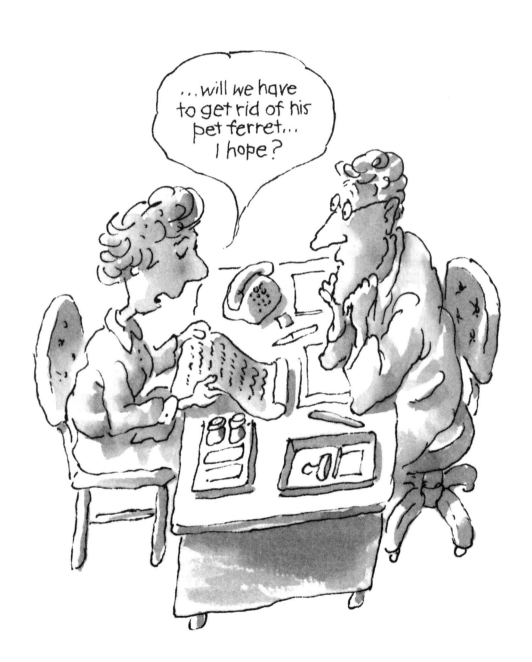

Chapter 7

Some questions that parents ask

When the diagnosis of asthma is made, parents are often apprehensive about what this means both for the present and the future. They may ask their doctor a few questions but often will realize, once they have gotten home, that there are a lot of other things they would like to have asked. They should be encouraged to return and see their doctor on several occasions to discuss their feelings and concerns in more detail. Don't be embarrassed to go to the doctor with a written list of questions. This chapter will deal with a few questions that the parents ask quite often but does not attempt to cover all the possibilities.

My child is 11 months of age and has just had a bout of wheezing after a bad cold. Does he have asthma?

After just one episode one cannot be sure. If you, his parents, or his older brothers or sisters have asthma, eczema or hay fever (i.e., are an atopic family), then it is certainly a possibility. On the other hand, he may just have had an episode of bronchiolitis, which is a viral infection leading to wheezing, which occurs in the first year of life. Time will tell if he is going to develop asthma; if he has recurrent episodes of wheezing, then he has asthma.

My three-year-old child often has chest trouble. My doctor says that he has wheezy bronchitis. Is that right?

The term wheezy bronchitis is a rather loose one and often such children have asthma. It is probably better to say that the child has asthma and to explain what this means. Children with 'wheezy bronchitis' will almost always respond to the medicines used for the treatment of asthma rather than the antibiotics which are so often prescribed.

My daughter, age seven, coughs a lot, especially at night. My doctor has given me cough medicines and antihistamines with little effect. What should I do?

Recurrent coughing, especially nighttime cough, may be a symptom of asthma. Indeed it may be the only symptom. Your daughter should see a pediatrician who may arrange for pulmonary function tests or start her on a bronchodilator (e.g., slow-release theophylline). If the cough goes away with the medication, this supports the diagnosis of mild asthma.

My son, who is eight years old, likes to play football. When he has been running for a while he gets short of breath and wheezes. What should I do?

Your son almost certainly has exercise-induced asthma (see page 23). By giving him a bronchodilator such as Ventolin, or by using sodium cromoglycate (Intal) before he begins exercising, the wheeze will be almost totally prevented.

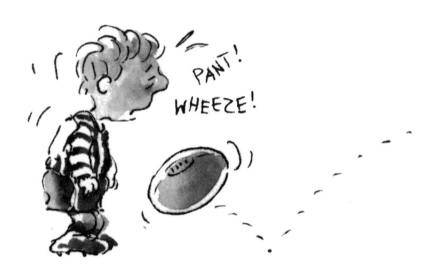

What activities should my asthmatic son avoid?

Probably none because of his asthma. The answer to this frequently asked question is one of common sense. The child will know what he can or cannot do. He should be encouraged to try everything and then, if necessary, limit his activities according to his capabilities.

My child has been taking TheoDur for the past month. My doctor wants to do a 'blood theophylline' test on him. What for?

Theophylline (aminophylline) is a medicine occasionally used in the management of asthma. Sometimes it can be quite difficult to find the right dose of theophylline for a child without their having a bit too much of the medicine. In these situations, it may be useful to check the blood theophylline level. This rarely needs to be done.

My child gets quite shaky and jittery after taking Ventolin. Is this normal?

Most of the bronchodilators have some central nervous system stimulant effect, to a greater or lesser extent. It is usually short lived and you will notice the child will be a little jittery, maybe slightly wide-eyed and hyperactive.

One of my friends swears by a special diet for helping her child's asthma. Should I give it a try?

There is no good evidence that food components induce asthma (see page 20). In general, patients who have food allergies will develop symptoms very soon after eating the food. Not only may they wheeze, but they will also get swelling of the eyelids, face, lips and maybe hands and feet. You may want to try the diet, but do not be disappointed if it does not work. Sodium metabisulfite, MSG or tartrazine can cause asthmatic attacks in susceptible patients, but usually this reaction is fairly obvious (see Appendix 1).

My neighbor's child has asthma and she had a lot of skin tests done. Should my asthmatic son have these done?

These are rarely of help in the diagnosis of asthma (see page 30). Often one will find multiple minor allergies on skin testing about which nothing can be done from a practical point of view.

My son has asthma and we have two dogs and a cat. Should we part company with our pets?

Pets are not commonly a cause of asthma. One way of finding out if the pet is part of the problem is to give the pet a vacation with a friend or in a kennel. If the asthma decreases greatly or ceases completely, then it may be necessary to part with the pet. This is rarely necessary.

Can asthma be cured?

As the basic cause of asthma is presently not known, it cannot be cured. However it is important to remember that the *vast majority of children* have a mild episodic asthma; most children will grow out of their asthma, and while it will not be cured, it will no longer be a problem for them.

My daughter is ten years old and she has had numerous asthma attacks since she was two years of age. Can this affect her heart?

No, childhood asthma almost never damages the heart and as she grows out of her asthma, her lungs will get back to normal. However you should remember that the hyper-reactive state of the bronchi remains. This means that she should be discouraged from ever smoking. Occasionally when exercising, she may have a mild attack of asthma, but this will respond rapidly to treatment.

Is asthma inherited?

As has been discussed in this book, some families are more 'atopic' than others. In such families there is a greater frequency of eczema, hay fever and asthma. So the tendency to develop asthma is, at least in part, inherited and is then modified by one or more of the factors shown on page 16.

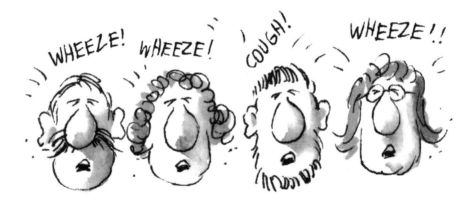

I have read about lung function tests in adults with asthma. Are they useful in children?

Yes they are. Young children, under the age of six or seven, may not be able to do them easily, but in the older child they are useful. You will remember that the problem in asthma is one of breathing out and lung function tests tell you how much air can be breathed out (exhaled) in a fixed amount of time. This gives an idea of how narrowed the bronchi are at that time. A simple mini–peak flow meter can be used by the older child at home to measure their lung function when required and this will help both you and your doctor in deciding on appropriate treatment.

My pediatrician has prescribed prednisone for my daughter who has quite severe asthma. Our neighbor takes it for arthritis and has had a lot of side effects. Is it safe for my daughter?

Prednisone is one of the oral steroid drugs. These are very effective in the treatment of acute asthma, although it is not understood exactly how they work. They are not bronchodilator drugs as such, but seem to reduce the swelling of the mucosa of the bronchi and also reduce the tendency for the smooth muscle in the bronchi to contract.

   Side effects may occur if oral steroids are used for prolonged periods. These include weight gain due to an increased appetite and retention of fluid, fullness of the face, an increased number of infections and a slowing of growth may also rarely occur. Side effects can be minimized by using oral steroids for as short a time as possible or in the child who needs steroids regularly by using the smallest dose. However in situations where steroids are used, the side effects of the asthma far outweigh the side effects of the medication.

There are so many medicines available for the treatment of asthma, which are the best to use?

You should discuss this with your doctor. Parents find that knowing when to give medicines by mouth as opposed to by inhalation is confusing. The difference is that when a medicine is given by inhalation it gets directly to the bronchi and so has an effect within a minute or two. Medicines taken by mouth have to be absorbed from the stomach and intestine and so do not have an effect for 30 to 60 minutes. This means that the choice as to how to give the medication depends on the severity of the attack. In the acute attack, it is better to give medication by inhalation first and follow this up with an oral (by mouth) dose. In the mild attack, oral medication may be quite adequate.

When should we use antihistamines?

They should never be used in an acute attack of asthma as they have a sedative effect, and this may be dangerous. They may occasionally be helpful in the child who has hay fever. In this situation they will help to dry up the running nose but will not have any particular effect on the asthma.

I have read about desensitizing (allergy) shots for asthma and hay fever. Are they worth trying in my son who has asthma?

While there are some children who seem to improve after a course of desensitizing injections, this form of treatment has not been shown to be really useful. Some children may improve after 'shots' which just contain water! A desensitization course is quite painful and is not without risk. Some children will get quite marked reactions like big insect bites at the site of the injection and very rarely there may be a much more severe reaction. Desensitization is not recommended in asthma. It may, occasionally, be useful in hay fever.

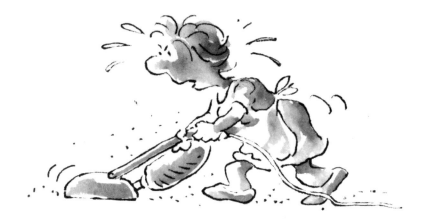

How can I make my house 'dust-free'?

Of course this is not possible. About 70 percent of children with asthma are allergic to house dust and in particular the house dust mite, although it is still unclear how important this is in causing asthma in children. The child's bedroom should be kept clean and as free of dust as is practical. Some parents will remove carpets from the bedroom and replace it with linoleum. Blankets should be washed regularly and putting a layer of polyethylene between the mattress and the sheet may be useful. However you should be aware that these measures may not greatly improve your child's asthma as other provoking factors may be more important.

My 40-year-old cousin who has asthma has found hypnosis useful. Would it be helpful for my ten-year-old son who also has asthma?

In general, hypnosis is of no value in childhood asthma. Very occasionally a child may be taught how to hypnotize themselves (auto-suggestion) and can abort an attack of asthma. This is quite an unusual event.

At what times of the day should I give my daughter her bronchodilators?

This obviously depends on the severity of her asthma. If her asthma is mild, she may be controlled with medication in the morning and the evening. If the asthma is more severe, she may need to take her medication to school with her. She can easily carry a metered aerosol (puffer) with her so that she can use it when necessary. Children do not like to be seen by their friends as having to take medicines; as a result they may tend to skip their midday dose of medicine. This is particularly the case during adolescence.

Negative ion generators are being heavily advertised. Are they useful in managing asthma?

With all the pollution that we live in, it is attractive to think that the air that we breathe in our homes can be 'purified.' At present there is no good evidence that negative ion generators are useful in the management of asthma. This does not mean that you should not try such a machine if you so wish. They are fairly expensive, so it might be wise to borrow or rent one for a while to see if it works before buying one.

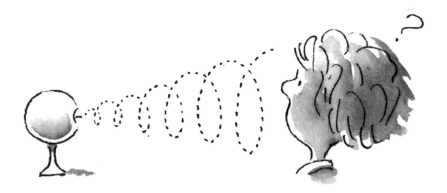

I am always worried that my son may have an asthma attack at school and that the schoolteacher will not know what to do.

Schoolteachers are not doctors or nurses and so do not claim to know too much about asthma or any other medical condition. However most schoolteachers will have children in their classes who have asthma and will have some experience of what to do. It is up to you as a parent to meet the schoolteacher or school nurse and let them know that your child has asthma. Provide them with information about your child's asthma:

- How often attacks occur.

- Is it brought on by exercise (exercise-induced asthma).

- Write down for them the medications that your child is taking and how often they should be given.

- If necessary, obtain an explanatory letter from your doctor for the school.

Most schoolteachers are given little information by parents and are then criticized for not 'acting correctly' when a problem arises. This is hardly fair on the teacher.

My son, who has quite frequent episodes of asthma, has been looked after by our general practitioner. I was wondering if it would be wise for him to see a specialist?

There is no black-and-white answer to this question. Often the general practitioner who knows the child and family well is the best person to deal with the youngster's asthma. Guidelines for seeing a specialist include:

- Frequent attacks of asthma that respond poorly to treatment.

- Chronic symptoms that do not go away.

- Recurrent attacks that stop the child from attending school.

- Attacks which are sufficiently severe to require the use of steroid medication.

These are purely suggestions and should be interpreted in a commonsense way. Some parents may feel the need to consult a specialist sooner than others.

Can other nebulizer solutions be mixed with Intal nebulizer solution?

Ventolin, Bricanyl and Alupent respirator solutions can be mixed with Intal in the nebulizer. If medicines are mixed in the nebulizer, they should be used soon after mixing.

My son has a Ventolin inhaler and it often runs out just when he needs it. How can I tell when it is nearly empty?

This is a frustrating problem. One way of avoiding it is always to have a second canister (refill) available. The other way of knowing how much is left in the canister is shown on page 73.

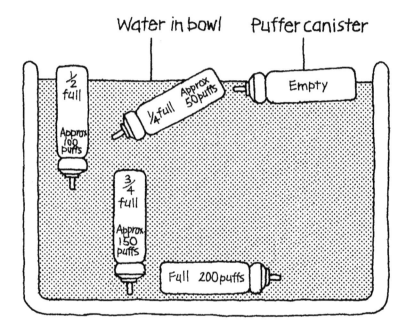

How much liquid is left in the canister? A simple test to measure how much is left in the canister is shown. A bowl is filled with water and the position the canister takes in the water indicates the amount remaining.

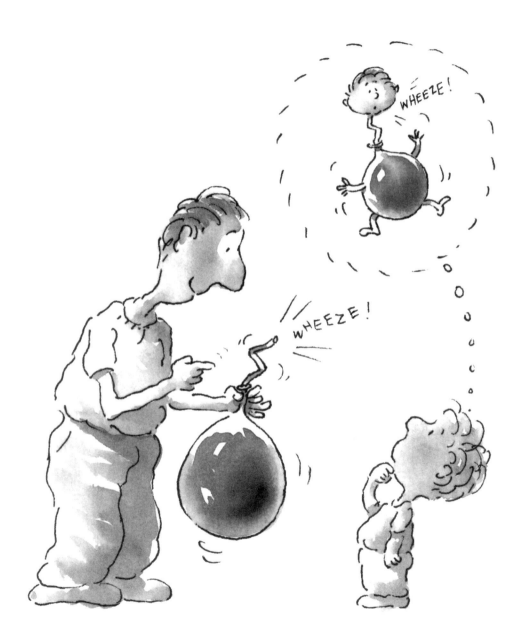

Chapter 8

Explaining asthma to young children

Young children may, and do, get asthma. For them it is a frightening experience and for parents it is often difficult to explain what is happening. It is hoped that when parents have read this book they may be in a better position to explain to their young child with asthma what is happening to him or her. Each family has their own 'domestic language' with which they speak to their children, so it would not be possible to write a chapter which would cover the needs of all families. It is best for parents to explain to children what is happening to them in their own way and this section outlines a few suggestions for parents to interpret in their own way.

• Use the word asthma to describe to your child what is wrong with him or her. It does not help to beat about the bush and use lots of other vague expressions. Many children, even when young, will know, or know of, another child with asthma. It may help them to understand better if they can relate to John or Sarah who also has asthma.

• Explain how air gets from the mouth and nose to the lungs, which can be described as balloons which go up and down as the air goes in and out. The air travels down the bronchi of which we have spoken before. Bronchi can be likened to drinking straws, long tubes through which the air travels. In asthma, the problem is that the bronchi are narrowed. This can be likened to a drinking straw which has been bitten or chewed and is narrower than usual. This makes it more difficult to drink through and less cold drink comes up the straw. In the same way, less air gets out of the balloons (lungs) because the bronchi (straws) are narrowed.

• Young children will not necessarily be concerned about wheezing as such. They are usually frightened because their breathing is noisy and because they feel that they cannot breathe normally. The noise is because the air is being forced through the narrowed straw. This can actually be demonstrated to the child by a parent blowing through a normal and a narrowed straw. The feeling of 'not being able to breathe' is because the air cannot get out through the narrow straw. This can be demonstrated by blowing up a balloon and showing the child that it empties more slowly through a narrow tube, or straw, than through a wider one.

• Coughing is quite common during an attack of asthma. This is because of the mucus in the bronchi which is being cleared.

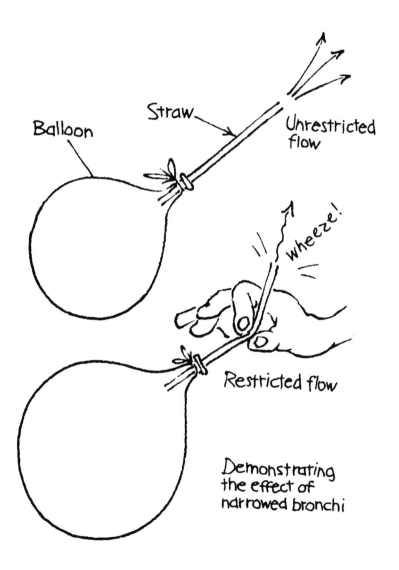

Balloon

Straw

Unrestricted flow

wheeze!

Restricted flow

Demonstrating the effect of narrowed bronchi

This may be explained by using examples of 'sticky stuff' like pudding, custard or some other sticky substance that the child is familiar with.

- Medicines need to be taken to make the asthma better. The medicines make the airways wider; in other words, it helps to make the straw wider, or better, again. For some children it may be appropriate to actually suggest that the bitten, narrowed straw is a 'sick straw' and that the medicines will make it into a 'healthy' straw again.

- Medicines may be given by mouth or by a nebulizer. Most very young children will not manage to take medicines in any other way. The medicines that go in the mouth are usually colored liquids and don't taste too terrible. They go into the tummy and then all over the body and will reach the 'narrow straws' to make them healthy again. The nebulizer is like a mask that a pilot wears in an airplane to help him or her breathe. Out of the mask will come a fine spray of water and medicine and that goes right down the straws to the balloons. This also will help to make the straws healthy again. Usually the response to the nebulizer is both good and rapid; this can be used to reinforce how useful this treatment is and with luck using the nebulizer can become a bit of a game. The child needs to know that the nebulizer will need to be used on several occasions before the straws are quite healthy again.

- It may be necessary for the child to be admitted to the hospital for a day or two. This is often made much easier these days as parents very often will stay with the child, if it is possible. Many children will just need regular sessions on a nebulizer, which is painless and can be made quite fun. In more severe cases, it may be necessary to put up a drip to give medication into the vein. This is always slightly uncomfortable as the needle is being put through the skin into the vein. Discomfort can be minimized by the parents being present and the doctors being friendly and chatty with the youngster. Once the needle is in, most children will settle down quite well, especially if they begin to feel that they can breathe more easily and are feeling better.

These are only suggestions as to how to explain asthma to the very young child. They are meant as a guide for parents to interpret in their own way.

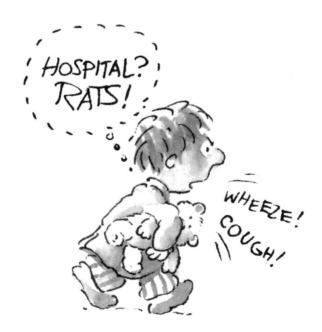

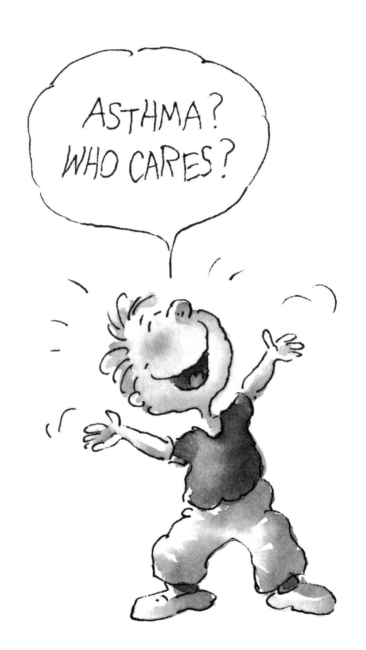

Conclusion

As has already been explained, asthma is a common problem in childhood. However it is very important for children and parents to realize that *for the vast majority of children it is a mild, although annoying, illness.* It should be seen more as an inconvenience, than as a disease which is going to interfere with the child's lifestyle and development. It is also very important to remember that while there is no 'cure' for asthma, present-day treatment is very effective with very few side effects indeed.

This book may have answered some of your questions about asthma; ask your doctor for more information about the condition itself and the medications. Try the asthma quiz on the next page and see how much you have picked up by reading this book.

Asthma quiz

	True	False	See page
1. The commonest event to provoke an attack of asthma is a viral infection.	☐	☐	17
2. Asthma is sometimes inherited.	☐	☐	15, 66
3. Pets are a common cause of allergic reactions.	☐	☐	20, 65
4. Night cough is common in asthma.	☐	☐	62
5. Sodium cromoglycate (Intal) is a *treating* medicine.	☐	☐	91
6. It is easy to know when the puffer canister is nearly empty.	☐	☐	73
7. Skin tests are useful in the diagnosis of asthma.	☐	☐	30
8. Asthma can be cured.	☐	☐	34, 65

	True	False	See page
9. Changes in diet are often helpful in asthma.	☐	☐	20
10. My eight-year-old son has asthma, so I should not let him play sports.	☐	☐	23, 54, 63
11. Every time my child goes to the hospital with asthma he needs a chest x-ray.	☐	☐	31
12. My nine-year-old daughter has frequent episodes of asthma. My doctor says that she should have a peak flow meter at home. Is that a good idea?	☐	☐	28, 50
13. My son who has asthma coughs a lot at night. I always give him cough medicine before he goes to bed. Is that right?	☐	☐	53, 62
14. Antihistamines are useful in treating asthma.	☐	☐	52
15. Slow-release theophylline (TheoDur) needs to be given four times a day.	☐	☐	92
16. Inhaled corticosteroids have as many side effects as when steroids are given by mouth.	☐	☐	91

	True	False	See page
17. Desensitizing (allergy) shots are useful in asthma.	☐	☐	52
18. Negative ion generators are useful in asthma.	☐	☐	55, 70
19. The condition of most children with asthma improves with age.	☐	☐	35
20. Today's medications for asthma are safe if properly used.	☐	☐	37
21. Antibiotics are useful in treating asthma.	☐	☐	62
22. In an attack of asthma, it is safe to use the home nebulizer every two hours.	☐	☐	59
23. In asthma, the airways are hyper-reactive.	☐	☐	12
24. In asthma, the lumen of the bronchi is widened.	☐	☐	12
25. Changes in the weather can cause an attack of asthma.	☐	☐	23
26. Food allergy is a common cause of asthma.	☐	☐	20
27. Asthmatic adolescents and adults may smoke.	☐	☐	21

	True	False	See page
28. Most asthmatic children are unduly nervous.	☐	☐	22
29. RAST testing is useful in the diagnosis of asthma in children.	☐	☐	31
30. Pulmonary function tests are uncomfortable for the child to do.	☐	☐	29
31. Episodic asthma is the commonest form of asthma in children.	☐	☐	34, 35
32. About 2 percent of children have severe chronic asthma.	☐	☐	34, 35
33. Wheezy bronchitis is best called asthma.	☐	☐	35
34. Episodic asthma needs maintenance treatment.	☐	☐	38

ANSWERS

1. T	7. F	13. F	19. T	25. T	31. T
2. T	8. F	14. F	20. T	26. F	32. T
3. F	9. F	15. F	21. F	27. F	33. T
4. T	10. F	16. F	22. F	28. F	34. F
5. F	11. F	17. F	23. T	29. F	
6. T	12. T	18. F	24. F	30. F	

Foods containing sodium metabisulfite, MSG or tartrazine

■ Sodium metabisulfite

Sodium metabisulfite is predominantly in acidic foods and beverages to prevent undesirable bacterial growth and food discoloration and to help maintain vitamin C in fruit juice. This preservative does not occur naturally. It is generally added to foods.

Asthmatic patients reacting to sodium metabisulfite develop a tightness in the throat together with wheeze within a few minutes of eating food such as a pickled onion or drinking a glass of white wine or orange juice.

■ Foods containing sodium metabisulfite

Beverages

Commercial chilled fruit juice with the exception of canned, pasteurized or aseptic drinks. Bottled drinks containing fruit juice.

Orange- or yellow-colored soft drinks in glass bottles
Cordials

Fruit

Dried 'tree' fruits such as apples, apricots, pears
Fruit bars

'Fresh' fruit salad from commercial outlets may have sodium metabisulfite added to maintain appearance.

Note: Sultanas, currants, and raisins do not contain sodium metabisulfite and prunes are not preserved with it.

Vegetables

Dried vegetables
Instant mashed potatoes
Pre-cut, pre-peeled or
    commercially prepared
    scalloped potatoes

Potato chips (inconsistent—
    some packets of chips do,
    others don't)
Pickled onions
Pickles

Meat, fish, poultry

Sausages
Hot dogs
Processed chicken

Processed cold cuts
Uncooked fresh prawns

Dairy products

Fruit yogurt

Cheese pastes

Miscellaneous

Vinegar
Goods containing vinegar such
    as salad dressings, sauces

Desert toppings
Flavoring essences
Jams

■ Monosodium glutamate (MSG)

Monosodium glutamate is a naturally occurring substance that is one of the building blocks of protein. In its natural form it is found in foods such as tomato, mushroom, fruit, corn and in cheese (parmesan, Camembert, blue vein). Apart from the three cheeses mentioned which have a high MSG content, MSG in its natural form is unlikely to cause a problem.

However, the majority of MSG in the diet comes from food to which it has been added as a flavor enhancer. There is consider-able evidence that MSG used as a food additive causes symptoms other than asthma in sensitive individuals. To avoid MSG in foods it is very important to read labels on food products very carefully and also to avoid foods labeled as containing hydrolyzed vegetable protein, added flavor and/or spices as these may also contain MSG.

■ Foods containing monosodium glutamate

Chinese, Japanese, Asian foods
Foods with the highest content
    of MSG are fried rice, foods
    with batter or crumbs and
    foods with spicy sauces
Take-out pizza, especially
    spiced or seasoned
Take-out seasoned chicken
Commercial savory foods
Packet or canned soups
Pies
Sausage rolls
Hot dogs
Canned and luncheon meats
Meat and fish pastes

Frozen prepared dishes
Canned vegetables in sauce
Flavored potato chips
Savory biscuits
Cocktail onions
Pickles
Soy sauce
Mixed seasonings and
    spiced seasonings
Gravy-makers
Stock cubes
Tomato puree, paste and sauce
Commercial breadcrumbs
Stuffing mixes
Yeast and meat extracts

■ Tartrazine (yellow food dye)

The yellow food dye tartrazine is the color of most importance to
asthmatics. This has been a well-known provoker of asthma for
many years. It can be found in foods, beverages, tablets, capsules
and medications.

■ Foods containing tartrazine

Medications colored yellow,
    green, orange
Commercial fruit juice
Cordials
Cookies
Pastries
Cakes

Desserts
Toppings
Syrups
Soft drinks
Packaged snack foods
Sauces
Pickles

Drugs used in the treatment of asthma

This is not necessarily an exhaustive list of medications available, but covers those most commonly used in childhood. The medications are listed in alphabetical order using their proper names with their brand names in parentheses. The reason for doing this is because more than one company may manufacture a product with the same basic ingredient.

Parents and older children should be aware of the dose of the medication prescribed and the possible side effects. Most bronchodilators have similar side effects, which occur rarely unless the medication is being used in excess (overdosing). These side effects are shakiness, nervousness, palpitations and headache. Inhaled medications very rarely produce any side effects, as little of the medication is absorbed into the bloodstream.

■ Albuteral (Ventolin)

Albuteral is a bronchodilator drug. It is available in these dosage formats: 4mg tablets, 2mg/5 ml syrup, 100mg/dose metered aerosol (puffer) and a nebulizer solution of 5mg/ml and nebules of 2.5 and 5mg. Ventolin is also available in the form of 200-micrograms Rotacaps for inhalation. Albuteral is mainly a *treating drug* but can be preventative for exercise-induced asthma. It usually needs to be given three to four times a day.

■ Beclomethasone dipropionate (Vanceril, Beclovent)

Beclomethasone dipropionate, an inhaled steroid, is available as a metered aerosol (puffer) of different strengths (50, 100 and 250 micrograms per puff) for the prevention of asthma. This is a *preventative drug* and not a treating drug. The medication is taken regularly two to four times per day at the lowest dose that controls the symptoms adequately. Side effects with low doses are minimal. With high dosage, weight gain, fullness of the face and, rarely, growth delay may occur.

■ Choline theophylline (Choledyl)

Choline theophylline is available in a 200mg tablet (containing 133mg theophylline) and a syrup containing 50mg/5ml (equivalent to 33mg theophylline). This medication is a *treating drug* and needs to be used four times a day; side effects are as for theophylline (see below).

■ Ipratropium bromide (Atrovent)

Ipratropium bromide is available both as a nebulizer solution and as a metered aerosol. It is mainly a *treating drug* and side effects are very uncommon. It is often added to other bronchodilators in the nebulizer to increase their effect.

■ Orciprenaline (Alupent)

Orciprenaline sulfate is available in several preparations: 20mg tablets, 10mg/5ml syrup, 15mg/ml metered aerosol (puffer) and both as a 2 percent and 5 percent inhalation solution for a nebulizer. Orciprenaline is mainly a *treating drug* and needs to be given three to four times a day.

■ Prednisone/Prednisolone (Pediapred, Prelone)

Prednisone and prednisolone are oral steroids, which are both broken down to the same active end product in the body. They are mainly used in patients with acute, severe asthma, when other medications have not been effective. They are strong *treating drugs*. Preparations are available as 1, 5 and 25mg tablets. They are usually given in 'short courses' lasting a few days, which keeps side effects to a minimum. Increased appetite is (probably) the most common side effect in this situation and is temporary.

In a few patients with severe, chronic asthma, prednisone may need to be given regularly (on a long-term basis). This is rarely necessary as most patients can be well controlled with inhaled steroids, which have less side effects.

■ Sodium cromoglycate (Intal)

Sodium cromoglycate is available as a 20mg capsule to be inhaled with a Spinhaler, a 20mg ampule of solution for a nebulizer or as a 200-inhalation puffer (1mg/puff) containing a liquid solution. It is a *preventative drug only* and is of no use in an acute attack of asthma. There are no side effects to speak of and the medication usually needs to be used two to four times a day.

■ Terbutaline sulfate (Bricanyl)

Terbutaline sulfate is a bronchodilator drug and is available in a number of forms including 2.5 and 5mg tablets, 3mg/10ml syrup, 0.25mg/dose metered aerosol (puffer) and a nebulizer solution of 10mg/ml. It is a *treating (reliever) drug* and needs to be given two or three times a day. It can be used in single doses before sports for the prevention of exercise-induced asthma.

■ Theophylline compounds (TheoDur)

Theophylline is a *treating drug* but when taken regularly in the slow-release form (TheoDur sprinkles) is also a preventative treatment. The slow-release preparations have the big advantage of only needing to be given once or twice daily as opposed to three or four times a day. Side effects of all these preparations are similar and include nausea, vomiting, shakiness, overactivity, anxiety, and headache in up to 20 to 25 percent of children. The dose should be adjusted according to the child's weight to minimize side effects.

Action or 'crisis' plans

After your child's asthma is diagnosed, your doctor should discuss what to do in any future attacks and provide you with a crisis (or action) plan: written guidelines to help you through possible emergencies. This should be individually written for each child and include the following details:

- when to start extra medication;
- how to increase it;
- how much you can safely give;
- when to call the doctor or go to the hospital for additional treatment.

Some plans also include the measurement of peak flow during the attacks as it can be helpful to monitor an older child's response to the extra treatment.

An *example* of a simple 'crisis plan' would be:

	Medicine	*Dose*	*How often*
Regular medication	Intal Spincap	1 cap	3x daily
If coughing or wheezing *add:*	Ventolin Rotacaps	1 cap	up to 6x daily
If cough or wheeze not improving *start:*	Ventolin nebulizer	0.5ml	up to 6x daily
If wheeze/cough *continues or gets worse*	Call your doctor or go to nearest emergency room		
Phone Numbers:	Doctor _____ Hospital_____		

North American asthma resources

United States of America

American Academy of Allergy
  and Immunology
  611 East Wells St.
  Milwaukee, WI 53202
  800-822-2762

American Lung Association
  1740 Broadway
  New York, NY 10019
  212-315-8700

Asthma and Allergy Foundation
  of America
  1125 – 15th St. NW, Ste. 502
  Washington, D.C. 20005
  202-466-7643

Mothers of Asthmatics, Inc.
  3554 Chainbridge Rd., Ste. 200
  Fairfax, VA 22030
  800-878-4403

National Heart, Lung, and Blood
  Institute
  P.O. 30105
  Bethesda, MD 20824-0105
  301-251-1222

National Jewish Center for
  Immunology and Respiratory
  Disease
  1400 Jackson St.
  Denver, CO 80206
  800-222-LUNG

Canada

Alberta Asthma Center
  Box 4033
  Edmonton, Alberta T6E 6K2
  403-492-9564

Allergy/Asthma Association
  208525 – 11th Ave. S.W.
  Calgary, Alberta T2R 0Z9
  403-263-7551

Asthma Society of Canada
  130 Bridgeland Ave., Ste. 425
  Toronto, Ontario M6A 1Z4
  416-787-4050

Canadian Lung Association
  1900 City Park Dr., Ste. 508
  Gloucester, Ontario K1J 1A3
  613-747-6776

Index

Other child-rearing books that can help . . .

There Is a Rainbow Behind Every Dark Cloud
Edited by Gerald G. Jampolsky, M.D.
An incredible book about overcoming fear, written and drawn by
11 kids facing life-threatening illness. Ages 7 to 13. 96 pages

Advice to Doctors & Other Big People from Kids
Foreword by Gerald G. Jampolsky, M.D.
A kid's chance to be heard in the world of health care.
Ages 7 to 13. 112 pages

Feelings: Inside You and Outloud Too
Barbara Kay Polland, Ph.D.
"An important book for parents seeking a bridge between their
own and their children's feelings."—*San Francisco Chronicle*
With easy-to-read text and over 40 black-and-white photographs.
Ages 4 to 8. 64 pages

The Parenting Challenge: Practical Answers to Childrearing Questions
Barbara Kay Polland, Ph.D.
A reassuring, common-sense guide for families with infants to 12-
year-olds. 232 pages

It's OK to Be You: A Frank and Funny Guide to Growing Up
Claire Patterson. Illustrations by Lindsay Quilter
"This sound, sensible guide catalogues some of the physical and
psychological changes kids can expect during puberty."
—*Publisher's Weekly*
Ages 8 to 12. 70 pages

Available in bookstores or order direct from the publisher.
For ordering information or a free catalog, call (800) 841-2665.

Tricycle Press • P.O. Box 7123 • Berkeley, California 94707